THE SCOLIOSIS CURE

Lawrence DelRe, D.C.

Publisher: Health-1st
20 Bailey Avenue, Suite 300; Pittsburgh, PA 15211

1-800-340-4823

info@health-1st.com

First Printing 2014

The Scoliosis Cure

It was 1985. There I was, a brand-new chiropractor in my equally new chiropractic office. Some very old friends were in my office with their six year old son. He had scoliosis, and it was severe. The projections for the degree of curve he had at that age destined him to be a "hunch-back" by the time he was eighteen years old. He was in my office for back pain and headaches.

Of course, he could end up in a body cast. He could also have metal rods implanted in his spine, perhaps cutting again to replace them as he grew. As you can imagine, this is an awful answer. Wherever the ends of those rods "stopped," the vertebral joints would be beaten and worn, doing the work of bending for the entire spine. The "rod area" of the spine would become like a fossil, or a rock.

After working on him, the headaches and back pain went away. However, every time Joey came in, I would do a quick check on his scoliosis "progress" by simply having him stand in front of me while I was seated, and I would check the levels of the tops of his shoulders. One was always at least an inch lower than the other. After two months, I gave up on the scoliosis and released him from active care.

I didn't want to leave the parents with nothing, so I designed a balance board with a golf ball on the bottom center to produce a balance board. They didn't exist then so I had one made.

I also told the dad to get a 6x6 piece of lumber and make a balance beam. I did these things because I had read research that indicated that scoliotic children had deficits in their "3D" sensory feedback loops. Their bodies apparently did not know that their spines were curving. The devices couldn't hurt, and might help. A trampoline might help, too. I think it would be worth trying.

I also did one other thing. I looked in an obscure book that has been lost over time. I believe it was written by one of two doctors: Applied Kinesiology founder George Goodheart, D.C., or Major Bertrand DeJarnette, D.O., D.C.
I think it was Dr. DeJarnette, the founder of S.O.T., but the group that carries on his work can't find the exercise that I found within that book. I don't remember the book's name.

So I've named the exercise: "The Scoliosis Exercise".

About two months after I released Joey from active care, my wife and I were driving out in the country, and decided to drop in on our friends. Well, no sooner was I on the sofa when little Joey came running up, and ask me to check him.

I sighed, and told him to turn his back to me, (so I could view my failure once again,) but lo and behold, his shoulders were absolutely level!

Shocked, I asked him to take his shirt off. Viewing from the back, his spine looked straight to me. I had him bend over for the standard scoliosis check, and very little "humping" was evident.

I happily told him, "Keep doing your exercises!" And so he did. Just about every day of every year.

When Joey was in high school he told me, "You know, if I start to skip my exercises, I'll see my shoulder start dropping in the mirror when I brush my teeth."
I told him he should keep doing the exercises until he stopped growing, (about eighteen years of age.)

1

Well, Joey is in his mid-thirties now, and he stopped in my office a few years ago. We had x-rays taken, and you would never know he had scoliosis at one time. He told me that he stopped using the "devices" after the first couple of weeks, and only used "The Scoliosis Exercise" during all those years.

Twenty Five Years Later:

A couple of years ago, another couple, friends of ours, had a son who was having spinal problems, and they brought him in to my office. We had x-rays done and found a scoliosis. He was twelve years old at the time. Unlike Joey's "nice" smooth "S" curve, this curve was "jerky", with relatively sharp turns to the left and right, due to some type of childhood injury.

Let's call him A. I gave him the Scoliosis Exercise. I still see him periodically, mostly doing soft-tissue work and monitoring his progress.

When A first started two years ago, his upper back, above the shoulder blade, on the right side, "humped" up a bit, while laying on his stomach. That went away in the first few months. He has been mostly "flat" and symmetrical when laying face down on my table since then. I always ask him about his diligence in doing his exercises, and remind him to keep it up.

This past summer, however, I was alarmed to see his left mid-back humping up, two visits in a row.

I was afraid we were losing control of the scoliosis. When I expressed my alarm and asked about the exercises, he told me that he hadn't been doing them much at all the past couple of summer months. I expressed strongly that his spine was now curving, and I didn't know if it could be stopped. I also told him that he would be shorter because of it. I had to get his attention.

The next time I saw him, (a month later,) he laid face down on the table and his back was flat and symmetrical again! I asked about the exercises and he said he had been doing them regularly again. He'll have to do them until he stops growing. A couple minutes a day is all it takes.

So what is it?

It is a "cross-crawl" exercise.

THE SCOLIOSIS EXERCISE

First: <u>Find the side of the weak psoas muscle:</u>

Looking at the image on the right, it is easy to see how a weak psoas muscle on one side, and a strong psoas on the other side could pull the spine one way or the other.

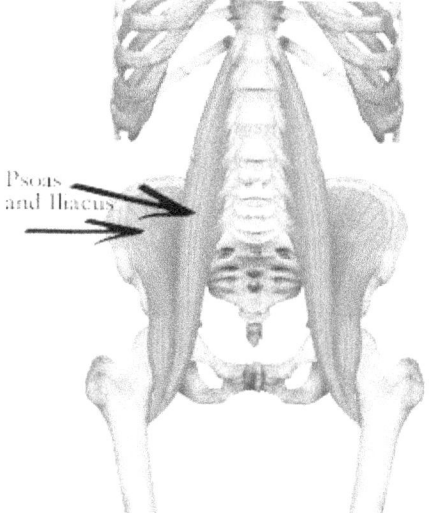

<u>Helper Method:</u>

- Have the subject lay on his/her back. Bring one straight leg up 45 degrees.
- Then take it out sideways 45 degrees.
- Point the toes outwards.
- Stabilize the pelvis by holding the opposite side of the the pelvis down, holding at the front top of the bone.
- Press the ankle that is up in the air, downward and outward by 45 degrees, telling the subject to resist.
- Get a feel for the resistance because this is the hard part if you haven't done this before.

Then do the same for the opposite leg. Figure out which side is the weak side. If you don't get it the after the first few tries, try again in a couple of hours, or the next day. It is very important to get it right.

When you know for sure which side is the weak side then the subject is ready for the exercises.

<u>Alternative method</u> of finding the weak Psoas muscle:

Subject lays on back. Bring both straight legs up 45 degrees, and then out 45 degrees, toes out. The subject holds this position until he/she can note which leg wants to drop more with exhaustion of holding it up. That is the weak psoas side.

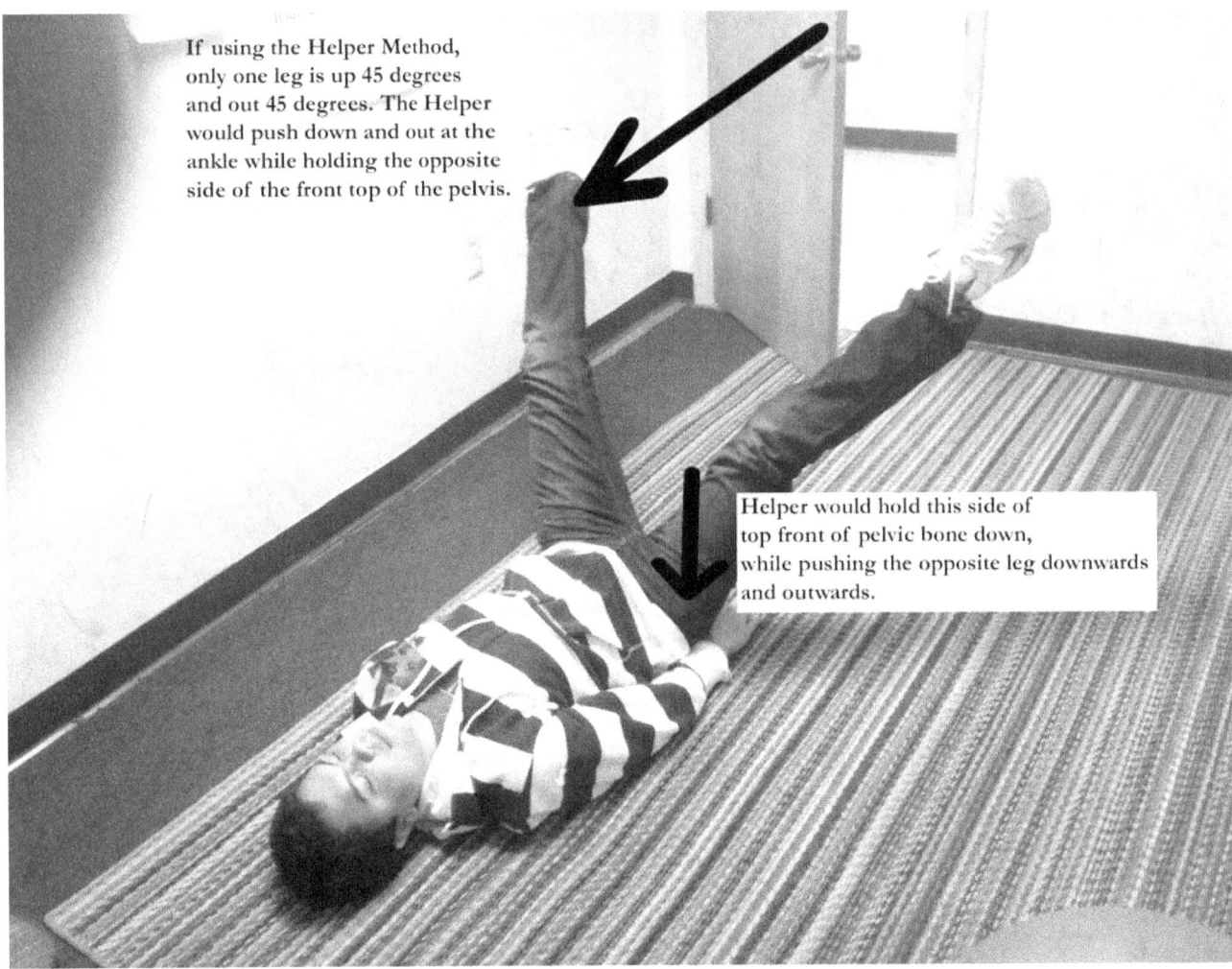

If using the Helper Method, only one leg is up 45 degrees and out 45 degrees. The Helper would push down and out at the ankle while holding the opposite side of the front top of the pelvis.

Helper would hold this side of top front of pelvic bone down, while pushing the opposite leg downwards and outwards.

The Scoliosis Exercise

Let's say the weak side of the psoas muscle is the left side.

The subject lays on his/her back, and "marches" with straight legs and arms, while laying on his/her back. Left arm goes up when right leg goes up, and vice versa. Simple. Don't complicate it. Bring each leg up high.

If the left psoas muscle is weak, think "left arm". Yes, "left arm". When "marching", while the left arm is up, the subject's head should turn to the left.

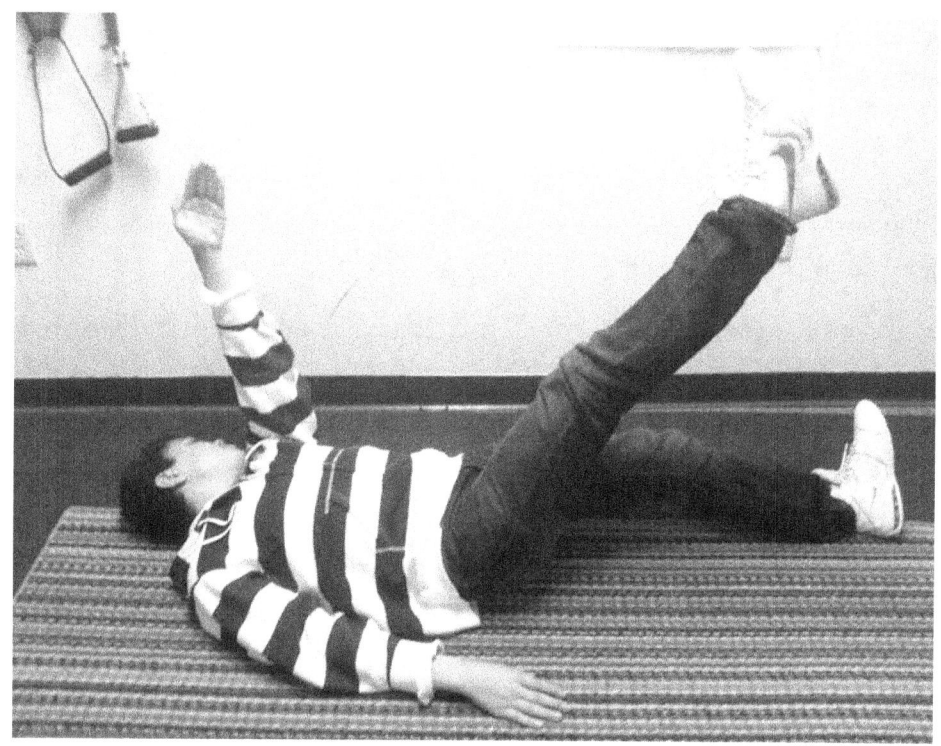

In the above picture, the subject's head is turned to the left for a weak left psoas muscle.

When the right arm is up, the subject's head goes back to center:

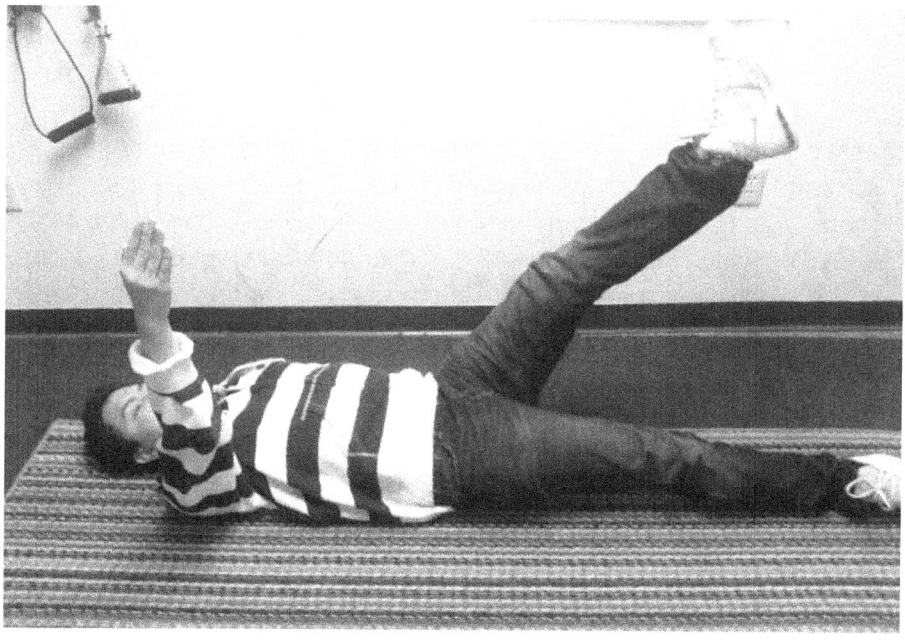

When the left arm is up, head goes left.

When the right arm is up, head looks straight up.

Start with ten repetitions per day. If you get sore, take a break for a day, then continue. Slowly increase to twenty reps per day. Thirty should be the maximum you need. A minute or two is all it takes. Unless there is pain, try to do them daily.

Will it work on everybody? I believe it will have a positive effect on most of those who use it, and may even be a complete cure, as in Joey's case. Because of Wolf's law, once a child is beyond eleven or twelve, it becomes exceedingly difficult to come to a complete cure.

I believe I am a responsible parent. Certainly before I let anyone cut on my child, I would have him/her use this exercise.

Progress

Progress can be judged by simply "eyeballing" the level of the child's shoulders after a month, and each month thereafter.

Also, the Helper can stand behind the child's back and lower his/her head to the child's height as the child bends forward to touch the toes. Look for a "rise" on one side or the other of the back. Look for the "high side", and write notes in the back of this book. Perhaps take an "un-selfie". That was a joke – take a picture with your phone.

Adults:

I have found that this exercise may help adults who have chronic low back pain - both with those with scoliosis and also those without scoliosis. If you test yourself and find a significant weakness on one psoas muscle, then you are a good candidate. It won't straighten your spine, but it may help.

Be careful! If you have scoliosis, you will have compensations built into your spine, and you will be balancing the muscles of the foundation of the spine. You will be changing things. This can have repercussions all the way up to your neck and base of the skull. If you experience back or neck pains, don't give up - just take a break. Use common sense and stop until any pain goes away. You have been like this all of your life and there is a lot of "defense physiology" built up in the muscles of your entire spine. A young child may need to do this exercise for his/her whole young life, until eighteen years of age, or longer. You, on the other hand, may only need to use it for a year or so, with occasional "tune-ups". You've got to think long-term with this exercise.

It would help to have someone do the same soft-tissue spinal massage I use in my clinic. I show how to do this on a YouTube video, this is Part 1 of a two part series:

http://youtu.be/PcLJ6GLL_Cc

---:

The only reason I am charging any money for this booklet is so I can pay Adwords to advertise it to the public. This is a work of charity I guess, because my plan is to put any money collected back into Adwords advertising in order to spread the message of this important approach to the deforming results of scoliosis.

If it works for your child, please help others by purchasing a number of books on Amazon - to give to your local orthopedic surgeons, physiatrists, and family doctors.

You are also permitted to copy this book, as much as you need, to reach others.

NOTES ON PROGRESS

You may want to use these pages for keeping track of exercise date completions.
It's best if the parent signs off in the beginning, and is encouraging.

Date	Signature	Notes

Date	Signature	Notes

Date	Signature	Notes

Date	Signature	Notes

Date	Signature	Notes

Date	Signature	Notes

Date	Signature	Notes

Date	Signature	Notes

Date	Signature	Notes

Date	Signature	Notes

Date	Signature	Notes

Date	Signature	Notes

Date	Signature	Notes

Date	Signature	Notes

Date	Signature	Notes

Date	Signature	Notes

Date	Signature	Notes

Date	Signature	Notes